The Joy of Laser

Volume 2:
Launch Your Rental Revenue!

Dr. Youkey

DEDICATION

Thank you to every Laser owner who invested in the rentable Lasers to help the pets in the comfort of their own home. This booklet was written for you, to help launch your rental Laser business.

I would also like to say a huge thank you to J. Mark Strong who recruited me into the world of Laser therapy. Your guidance, knowledge and passion for this industry has influenced me to no end. I don't know of another person who works as hard as you do both nationally & globally!

And what would life be without the love & support of my life partner? Thank you for all that you do, so that I can concentrate on my passion for this industry. I couldn't think of a better partner to go through life with - thank you!!

Finally, to all the pets & animals who continue to inspire me - you make me want to help ease your pain. Your unconditional love is treasured.

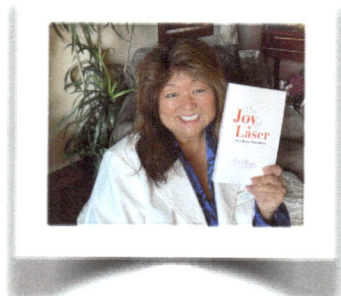

I thank you all and Happy Lasering!

Dr Youkey

WHY READ THIS BOOKLET?

Are you ready to launch you rental Laser business? Would you like some tips to fast track this new revenue source? For those who own other manufacturers' Laser, you can still get some great tips on how to generate income using rentable Lasers.

BENEFITS FROM THIS BOOKLET:
* Learn which Lasers make the best rentals
* Reveals valuable easy to implement ideas to market your Laser rentals
* On request, this booklet comes with a sample rental form that you can customize with your hospitals information
* Make money fast & launch your rental business to new heights - by using these techniques with any rentable Lasers
* A gift certificate applicable for future Lasers is included with the purchase of this book.

This is not a book explaining the theory of Laser therapy as there are plenty of resources already available. Instead, this book is a compilation of practical tips to launch your rental Laser business.

At the end of the book, there is a gift valued at more than the price of this booklet! This gift can be used on future Laser purchases with Dr. Youkey.

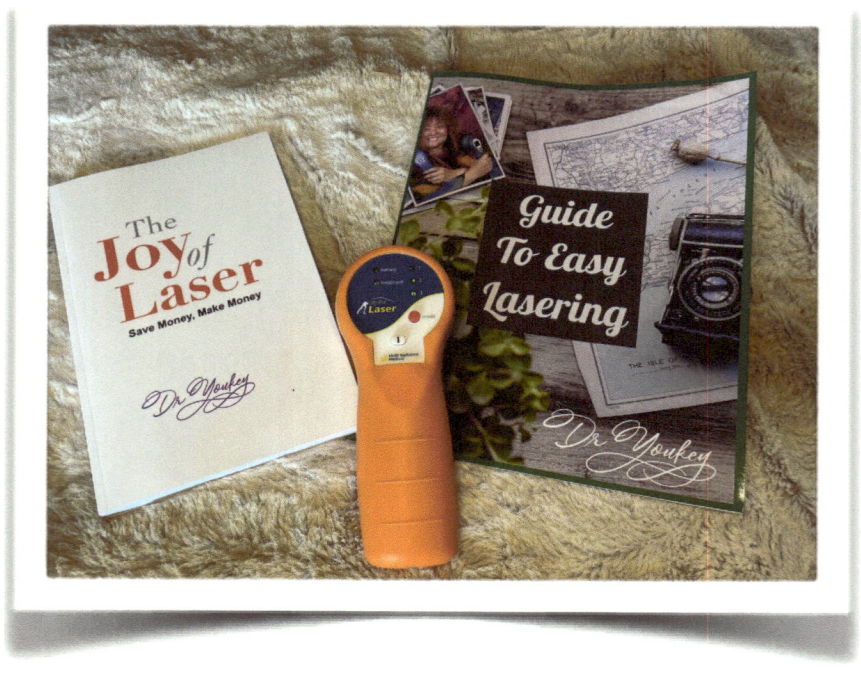

TABLE OF CONTENTS

DEDICATION	2
WHY READ THIS BOOKLET?	3
DISCLAIMER	7
WHY RENT LASERS?	8
CHOOSING A SAFE RENTABLE LASER	12
NOW WHAT!?!	18
HOW MUCH TO CHARGE	20
WHAT ABOUT INSURANCE?	23
USE RENTAL FORMS	25
PREPARE THE LASER	27
UTILIZE BROCHURES	29
UTILIZE FLYERS	31
ADVERTISING	32
CROSS PROMOTE	35
NEWSLETTER & BLOGS	37
CASE STUDIES & TESTIMONIALS	39
SUBMIT A PRESS RELEASE	41
CONTACT YOUR LOCAL RADIO & TV STATIONS	43
STAFF ENTHUSIASM!	46

CREATE DISCOUNT PACKAGES	48
IN-HOUSE RENTALS	50
SOCIAL MEDIA POSTINGS	52
WEBINARS & PODCASTS	55
INCENTIVES & REFERRALS	57
LOYALTY CARD	59
SPEAK AT LOCAL VENUES	61
AFFILIATE PARTNERSHIP	63
WANT MORE MARKETING TIPS?	65
BONUS OFFER	67
CONTACT INFORMATION	68

DISCLAIMER

Although the author and publisher have made every effort to ensure that the information in this book was correct at press time, the author and publisher do not assume and hereby disclaim any liability to any party for any loss, damage, or disruption caused by errors or omissions, whether such errors or omissions result from negligence.

The marketing tips revealed in this booklet have been used by other practicing physicians to launch their rental Laser business but in no way is meant to guarantee the success of your own business.

This book is not intended as a substitute for the advice of marketing professionals or physicians. The reader should regularly consult a physician in matters relating to his/her health and particularly with respect to any symptoms that may require diagnosis or medical attention.

The information in this book is meant to supplement, not replace, proper professional medical advice & care. Like any medical equipment, Lasers poses some inherent risk. The authors and publisher advise readers to take full responsibility for their safety and know their equipment and precautions necessary to prevent harm to the operator or patients. Before renting out any Laser, be sure that your equipment is well maintained, and do not take risks beyond the level of experience, aptitude, training, and comfort level of the renter.

Laser therapy should not be commenced until a diagnosis is reached and used only under the direct or indirect supervision of your physician.

Marketing ideas & suggestions presented in this booklet is solely from the Author. Not all the tips will apply to all situations.

Copyright © 2020 DR YOUKEY LASERRIFFIC

The contents of this book is copyrighted and all rights are reserved. No part of this book may be reproduced or transmitted in any form or by any means, electronic or mechanical, including photocopying, recording, or by any information storage and retrieval system, without written permission in writing from the author

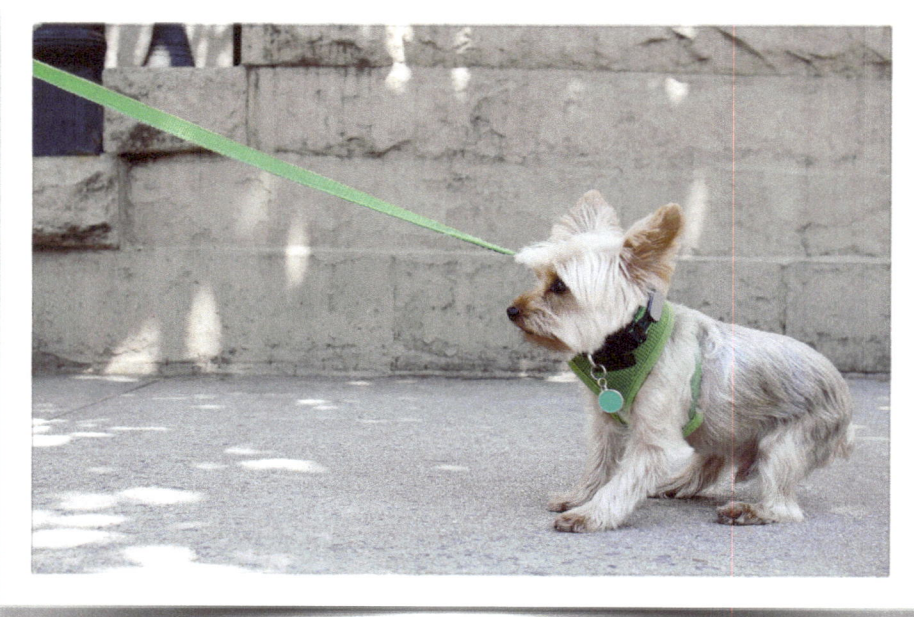

WHY RENT LASERS?

There are now safe, affordable FDA cleared Lasers available to send home with your clients. But what benefit can there be to invest in these Lasers? Why not have the client come into the clinic or hospital to receive their pets treatment?

There are a myriad of reasons to offer these rentable Lasers to your clients. Here are just a few:

1. Some pets just hate coming into the veterinary hospital.

2. Pets can get very stressed being around other scared pets. They can sense the anxiety from other pets & people too.

3. Some owners find it very difficult to return for repeated Laser treatments. Perhaps it is a physical challenge, transportation or lack of time available preventing them from returning for multiple sessions in a short period of time.

4. Reduces the risk of lost pets - if they run away during transportation to and from the vet.

5. Cats can finally receive the treatments they deserve. Many cats do not get the pain reduction treatments because of the stress induced by trying to get them to their vet.

6. Owners will experience less stress themselves by not having to transport their pets. This can mean less scratches, less muscle injury caused by big dogs pulling on their leashes, less anxiety for both the owner & the pets, and having to clean up less vomit, urine & feces in their vehicle (or carrier) from nervous or nauseous pets.

7. Pets get better treatment and more often with the owners giving the Laser sessions at home. This also means that the Laser treatments can reach the necessary dosage faster at home. Rather than 3 treatments in a week, the owner can give daily treatments to their pet, reaching faster results.

8. It can be more cost effective for owners plus they can treat multiple pets at home. I know many owners who have used the Laser on themselves, after seeing the pain relief in their pets.

9. Veterinarians can also resell the Lasers to their clients for chronic long term treatment needs. Dr. Youkey also offers an Affiliate Partnership Program to facilitate this.

10. Marketing materials, press releases, flyers and more are included with the MRM Lasers to help launch your service.

11. R.O.I. (Return On Investment) can be fast and many veterinarians will see a return on their investment in under 2 months!

12. Happy, healthy, pain free and stress free pets are the result of these amazing Lasers being used in the calm & comfort of their own home.

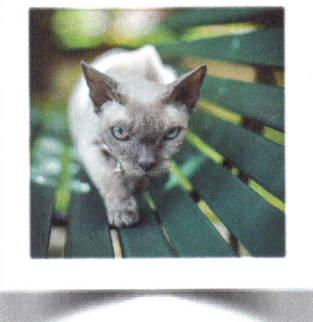

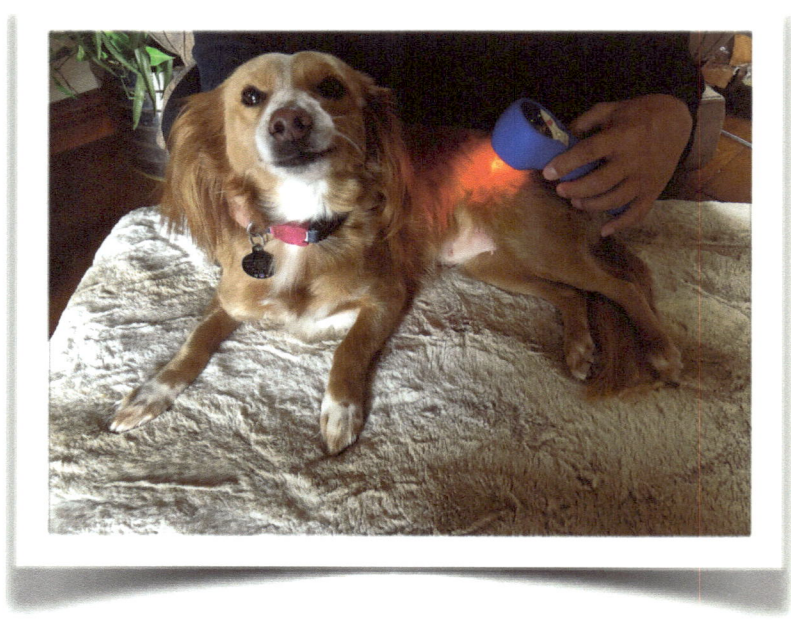

CHOOSING A SAFE RENTABLE LASER

Choosing which Laser to purchase is a huge choice. For those who have yet to choose their Laser, please ask for a Powerpoint presentation on "How To Choose Your Laser Wisely", from Dr. Youkey.

Remember that your license is on the line so be sure that the Laser you send home is both FDA cleared and is approved for use in the U.S.A. I couldn't imagine the liability from sending home a Laser that is dangerous enough to cause harm to any pet, person or property! Or sending home a Laser that is severely underpowered that does not provide the pain relief benefits as desired.

Listed below are some useful features to seek out when purchasing a Laser to use as a rental.

Features To Look For:

1. Make sure that they are FDA cleared.

2. Make sure that the Lasers are approved for use in the U.S.A. Inferior products may malfunction, generate a spark, or may not be compatible with the countries electrical capacity.

3. Be sure that the Laser has enough power to produce reliable reproducible results If the Laser is under powered (less than 1 Watt), the patient may not receive any benefit. The correct range of

frequencies and power is needed to produce a favorable outcome.

4. Be sure that the Laser has a variety of programs to choose from. The body gets used to just one frequency and it is better to change up, so the more choices, the better.

5. A cordless model is preferred over a corded one. Many cats and sensitive pets don't like having the cord brush against their fur. You also don't need to bring the pet near an electrical outlet if it is cordless.

6. Send only Lasers that are durable enough without many parts that can break such as the optical cord on a console unit. These parts (when out of the warranty period) can be very expensive to repair.

7. Use a Laser with the safest rating for rentals. Each Laser is classified from

Class I through Class IV. The higher the classification, the more potential for permanent retinal damage if used incorrectly.

8. A Class I does not need any goggles for the operator or the patient. A Class IV may require safety goggles for everyone between 5 - 20 feet depending on the Laser. This means everyone that comes into the area must have goggles on - the groomer, trainer, patient, other horses, goats, etc.

9. Never send home a Class IV Laser. That is a huge liability for you as these Lasers can permanently damage the eyes, and can even cause burns & fires if used incorrectly. And owners usually cannot comply to all the restrictions and regulations with the Class IV devices - such as blacked out windows & trip doors to stop the Laser if someone enters the Laser room, and many other

restrictions. Class IV are also banned at all outdoor equine events by USEF and FEI.

10. Class IV Lasers beep every few seconds to alert anyone within hearing range that the Laser is in operation that you must have goggles on. Class I Lasers do not beep like this, as there is no need for the warning. Sensitive patients don't like the beeping either. In some models, the beeping can be stopped.

11. Is the Laser backed by published peer reviewed studies and research? Some companies will use another company's study and pass it off as their own. Others continue to invest in research and studies to validate their own Lasers.

12. Ease of use is an important factor to consider when choosing a Laser to send home. It must be simple to use and must

not cause any harm should the operator make a mistake in their program choice.

13. Can this Laser withstand a dusty or humid environment? Some Lasers can be placed in a plastic bag such as a Ziploc® to protect the Laser from both dusty barns and rain.

14. Does the Laser have a blue light radiance to help combat bacteria, infections and MRSA? If you are sending home a Laser to combat these conditions, the 470nm Blue radiance has the most studies as an effective treatment.

15. Does the Laser have a long battery life? Some Lasers can be used for 50 treatments before needing a charge. So for short rentals under a week, you don't even need to send home the charger!

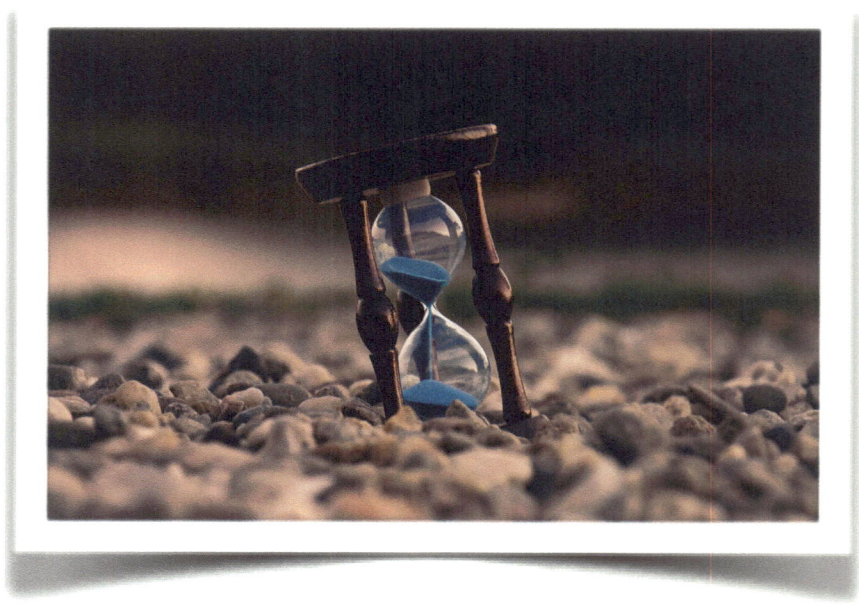

NOW WHAT!?!

Congratulations on your Laser investment! You are ready to start renting out your Laser. But now what!?! It's time to get to the meat of this booklet and show you some tips that you can easily use to help jump start your rental business.

If you purchased a Multi Radiance Medical Laser, you should have received a link to marketing materials filled with great resources. If you did not receive this, please ask Dr. Youkey for access at dryoukey@mac.com.

Each Chapter will highlight one of these marketing ideas. You choose which one to try out or all of them - you can determine how involved you would like to be. Some will work better in your particular situation and demographics than others. Most are totally free to employ and if you receive even one inquiry or rental because of your efforts - fantastic! But of course our goal is more than just one lead.

Remember that there are practices who are successfully renting out more than 30 Lasers on a consistent basis! I know doctors who invested in 20 of the rental units who is bringing in $25,000 a month revenue - so she retired! She is happy with that amount of income coming in, without having to do any of the work! Let's get you to that level with the tips on the following pages.

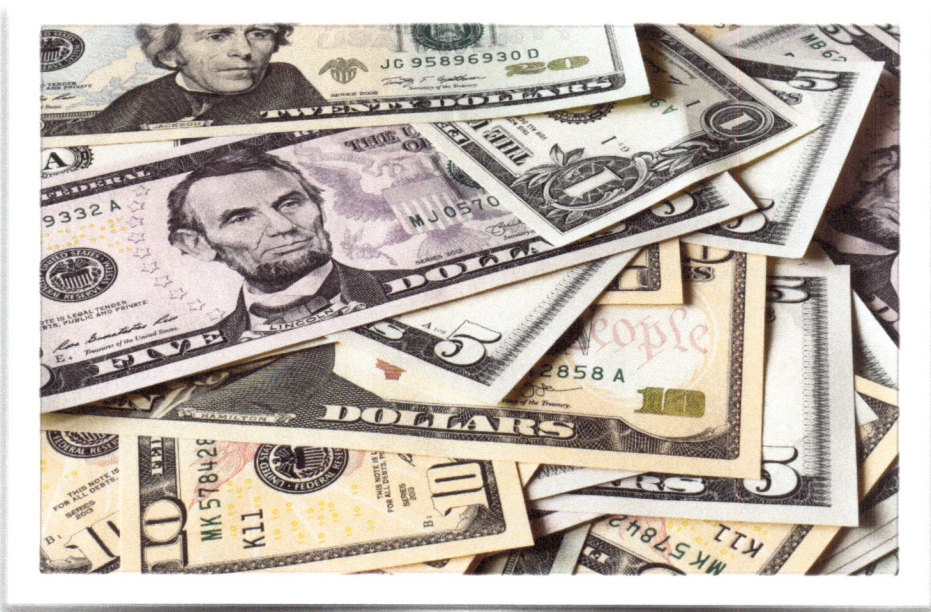

HOW MUCH TO CHARGE

There is no set amount to charge for rental Laser as this is different for all territories and demographics. Additionally, some physicians will charge per day, per week or per month. It is best to call around to various hospitals in your area to gauge the appropriate amount to charge.

It is not advisable to start with a lower amount and then expect to raise it later. It's best to start with the correct amount to begin with. Some hospitals will factor in how much they would have charged for the client to have the treatments done at the facility, compared to the savings of Lasering yourself at home. Usually there should be some savings factored in. Plus, the client can Laser all their pets or patients at home, so they are getting a very good value for choosing rental Lasers rather than coming back frequently to the facility.

As an example, I have seen rental Lasers range from $40 - $500 a week. Slightly more is charged for equine rentals versus small animal patients. Your R.O.I. will be faster if you charge appropriately.

Here is a worksheet from Multi Radiance Medical to calculate the amount you can generate with these Lasers.

Compare our ROI to any other modality!

Just one client rental / month creates substantial revenue!

With today's rising expenses and lost revenue to the Internet, it's a challenge to grow your practice net income. Let Multi Radiance prove how Laser rentals multiply quickly!

Your clients have been hearing about Laser's beneficial wound and rehab effects for years, but we are the only company offering you Class 1 safe and effective rentals for your clients.

Multi Radiance is committed to veterinarians

- ACTIVet PRO Laser System - Perfect for your practice
- Multiple MyPetLaser units - Perfect for client rentals
- Both come complete with Companion Protocol Manuals
- Complete Rentals Marketing Program to get started fast!
- Unlimited tech support for you and your techs

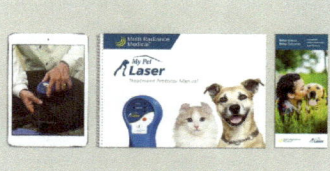

Great results for your client's pets
Great passive income generator for you!

Solve the problem of treatment consistency for arthritis, post-op healing, joint injury rehab, elder pet pain management, and lick granulomas. Add your clients to the rehab team! They love the convenience, cost effectiveness and safety of using our Super Pulsed Lasers in the stress-free comfort of home.

Go with the leader in Laser innovation with more peer reviewed studies than any other Laser therapy company. And we're practice proven with thousands of vets like you!

Rental Pro Forma Worksheet

MyPetLaser Rental Estimated Revenue Worksheet

	Practice Example	Your Practice
Number of patients seen per week	50	
% of patients with: pain, wounds, or are post-procedure	70 %	%
Patients with conditions that could benefit from stress-free, at-home laser	35	
Percentage that would qualify for rental agreement	25 %	%

Sample Laser Care Plan
 X Your Fee

Laser rentals per week	1	
Laser rental revenue per week	250	
Laser rental revenue per month	1000	
Laser rental revenue per year	12,000	
Total Laser Investment (one device)	2,500	

ROI is possible in 3 months or less

4 Weekly Rentals a month	6 Weekly Rentals a month	8 Weekly Rentals a month	10 Weekly Rentals a month
$12,000	$18,000	$24,000	$30,000

- Annual Passive Income -

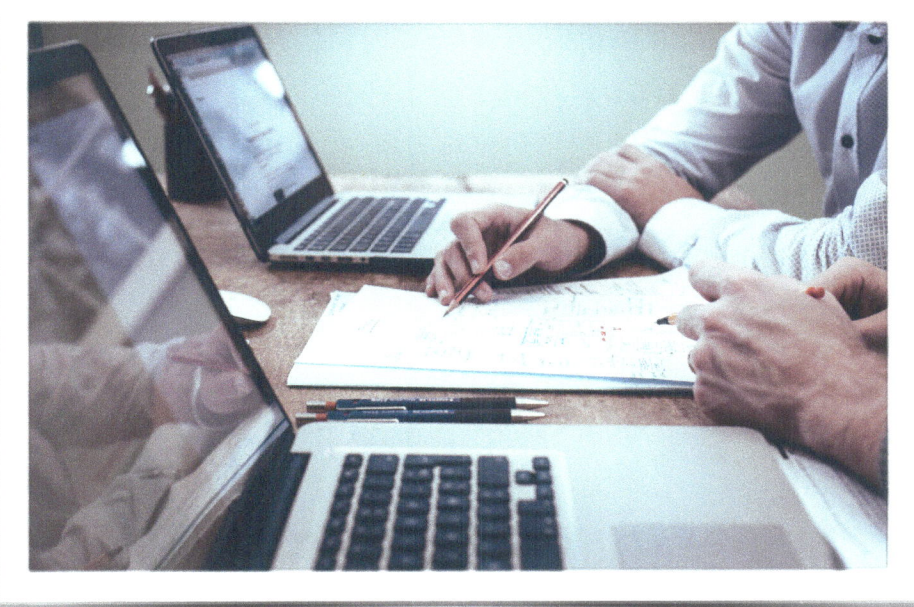

WHAT ABOUT INSURANCE?

Currently, 95% of the pet insurance companies will cover Laser therapy treatments performed by a veterinarian.

There are some pet insurance companies that will reimburse the owner for the cost of purchasing a Laser, if the veterinarian deems that the pet will need the Laser long term. Usually, this will require a prescription from their veterinarian and medical records to support the purchase.

Pet insurance companies will not cover Laser rentals. The owners will need to check their insurance policy to see what is covered. Usually, it is the middle plan that includes coverage for acupuncture that will also cover Laser Therapy sessions.

If the client were to purchase a package of Laser Therapy sessions and there is an invoice for each treatment performed by the veterinarian, the insurance may reimburse the clients.

An example of a package may be a bundle of six sessions at $50 each, for a total of $300 total.

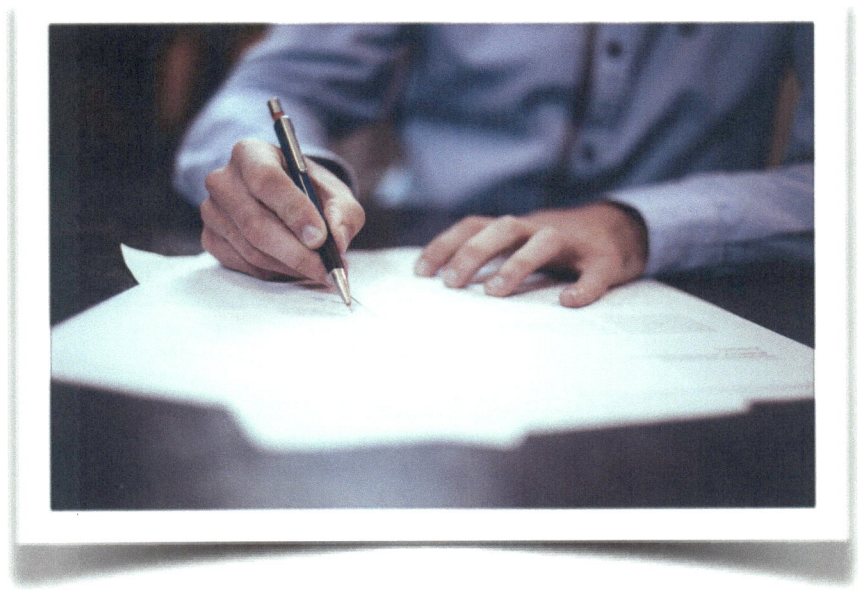

USE RENTAL FORMS

When you purchase a Laser from Multi Radiance Medical, you will receive marketing materials including rental forms to edit using your own hospitals' information. They are provided as either a Word document or PDF file. It is important to use these rental forms with each Laser you rent out. If you did not receive this form with your MRM Laser, contact Dr. Youkey for a copy at dryoukey@mac.com.

Some rental forms will have an area to note a deposit. It is wise to require a deposit for the amount of the Laser, should the medical device not be returned in the same condition as it left the hospital. This deposit can also cover lost chargers. You return the deposit once the Laser is returned in satisfactory condition.

Some owners will want to keep the Laser rather than returning it. This is when you can sell your Laser and keep the deposit. Contact Dr. Youkey for a replacement Laser at a special price.

If you purchased a Laser from a different manufacturer, ask the representative if they provide a Rental Form. Companies who sell FDA cleared Lasers for rental use should provide this legal document to protect you, your practice and your Laser.

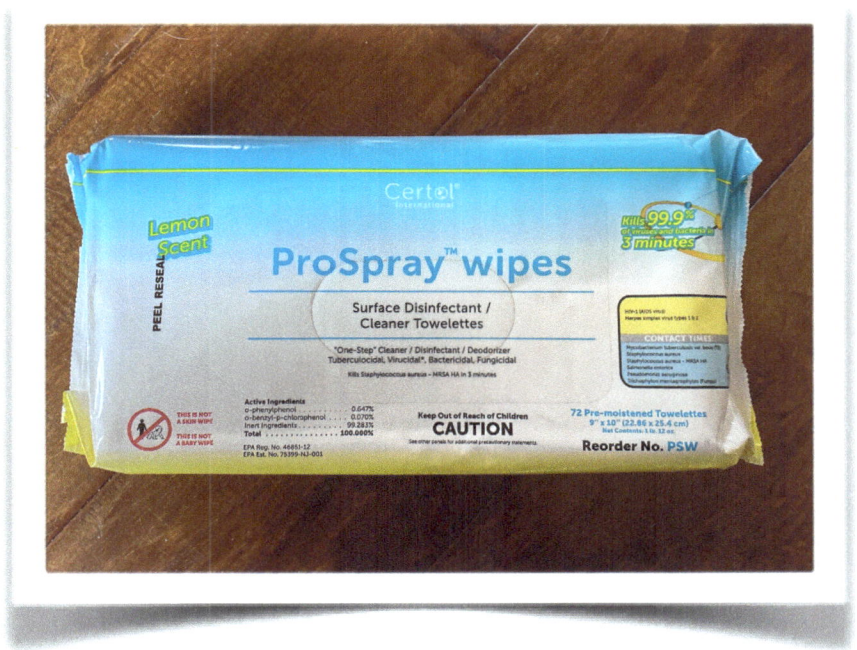

PREPARE THE LASER

Before you send the Laser to your client, be sure to charge it fully. Many owners will appreciate a fully charged Laser, rather than having to charge it before using the Laser.

Include the instructions and operational manual that came with the Laser. It is suggested make photo copies of the manual and send that with the client. Original manuals may be misplaced or damaged and is expensive to replace.

Be sure to clean and sterilize the Laser before renting it out. There are many ways to clean the Laser but the best medical grade plastic disinfectant wipes are called Certol. They can be purchased from any medical distributor. Follow the directions on the wipes for proper sterilization.

For infectious cases, you may want to remove the silicone rubber sleeve. The silicone rubber adds a nice tactile non-slip surface to grip, but makes it harder to clean.

Make sure to also clean under the silicone sleeve as well. Dirt and grime have a way of creeping in below the edges.

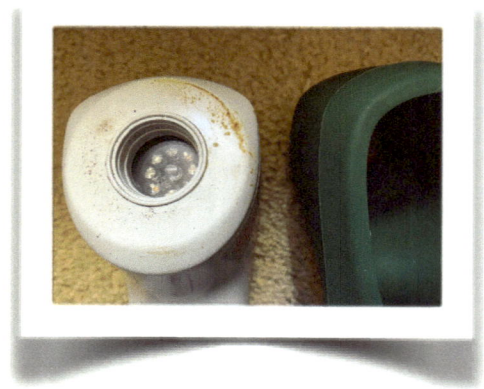

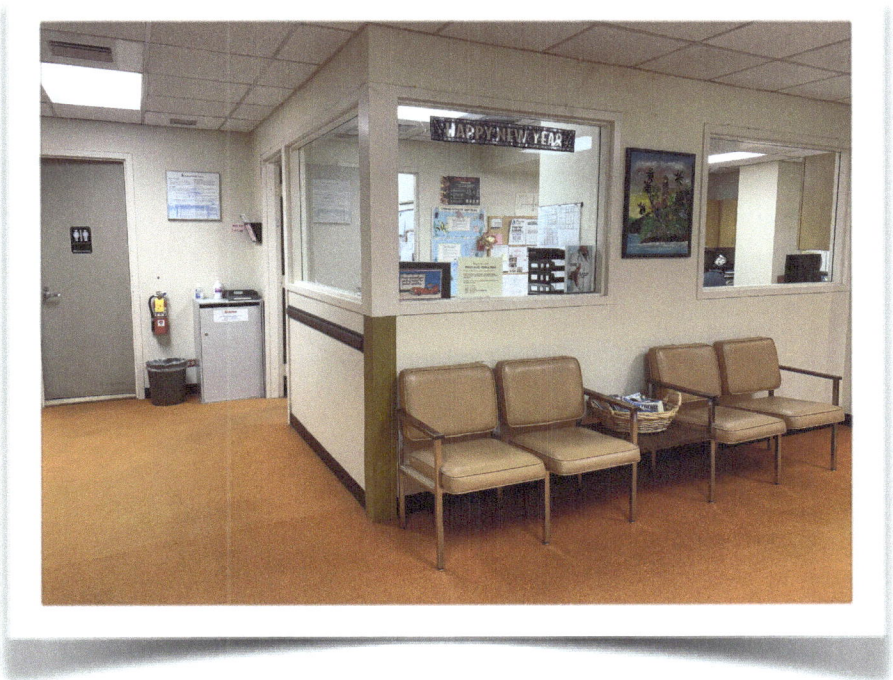

UTILIZE BROCHURES

Utilize the tri-fold brochures that your Laser manufacturers have already created. They help explain how Lasers work and also promotes Laser rentals if you have them displayed in the waiting and / or exam room.

Brochures advertising your rental Lasers is key to marketing your rental business. Let your clients know that you have this service available. Rather than your clients reading only magazines, leave brochures that will help advertise your practice services. Send these brochures home with your clients as they leave - along with their discharge papers.

MRM makes them available for purchase in packs of #100 but you can also create your own brochures using any word processing software. Ask you Laser manufacturer for their available brochures.

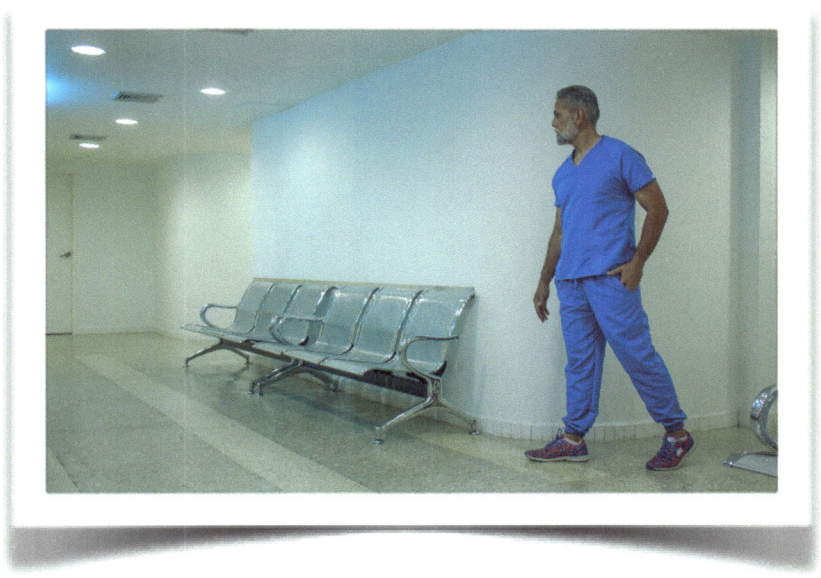

UTILIZE FLYERS

Some of the Laser manufacturers also provides flyers & posters to post in your exam room. This is effective silent advertising while your clients are waiting to be seen.

Utilize that valuable marketing space and place informational posters that will generate income for your practice. Contact your representative who you purchased your Laser from, to inquire about these free marketing materials.

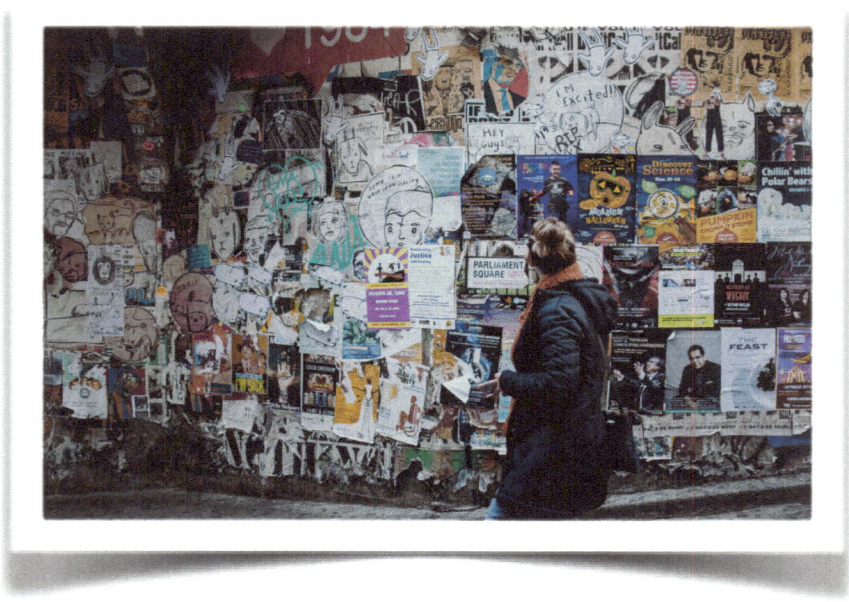

ADVERTISING

The world of advertising has shifted from the printed telephone books to more online presence such as Facebook banners. As an example, you can boost a posting on Facebook and pay per click on your business page. Print advertising still exists as display ads in national magazines, trade magazines, veterinary periodicals, newspapers and neighborhood magazines. As well as classified ads on your state veterinary websites.

Email is a tricky campaign. It's perfect for your current clients who have already opted in. But new regulations prevent you from sending emails to people who have not given their permission. So creating a funnel from your website or practice where clients can opt in - to receive your emails or newsletters. An iPad or other device like this in the waiting room is a great way to collect more emails as well as a check box on the admission papers.

Some veterinarians try direct mail advertising as well, sending letters to area pet owners. You can purchase these addresses but be sure that they are legitimate lists and guarantees a percentage of deliverable targeted contacts. Use a low cost printing company such as Vistaprint rather than expensive quick turn around places like Fedex Office Printing. Postcards will also save money compared to regular letters in postage. You can also purchase a list of new movers into your area which can be targeted for pet owners.

Car magnets are also an inexpensive way to advertise your new rental Lasers. Many companies can create an eye catching magnet with your logo and services on it. Just be sure to clean the car of any debris before putting the magnet on. And if you don't want a permanent fade mark on the paint finish, be sure to take it off occasionally.

Provide a coupon on businesses such as Groupon, Entertainment or a discount membership club such as Pet Assure. Although be aware that sometimes you may not make as much profit when participating in these venues. Read the fine print to make sure that your discount is not too steep - which may end up costing you money to offer the service.

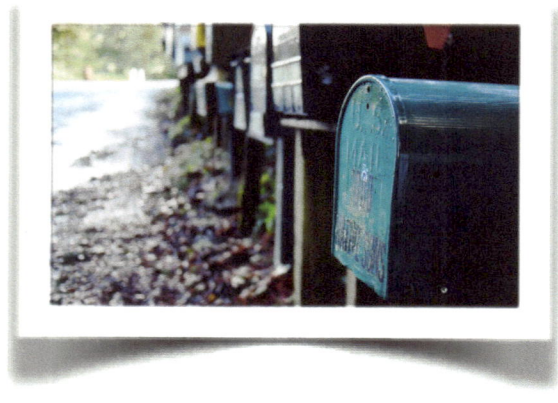

Post coupons on bulletin boards at local businesses and conferences. This may be an inexpensive way to get the word out about your service.

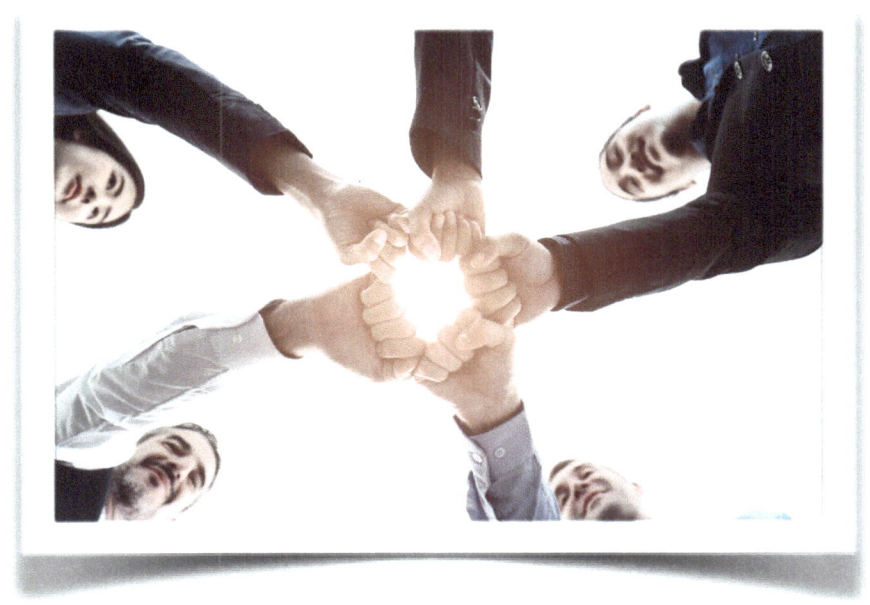

CROSS PROMOTE

Cross promoting your service with another existing business is a great way for both to prosper. For example, if a nearby hospital is not offering Laser services, approach the Practice Manager to work out an amicable deal. Perhaps you can refer clients back for services that you do not provide, in return for their referral of Laser therapy services through you.

This can also work with other types of businesses, by cross promoting your services on their website. In turn, you will also advertise their business on your resource page as well. Others have offered a discount to the staff of the cross promoting business to sweeten the deal.

The goal is not to steal any clients away, but to extend the services available for the best treatment modalities for the health of the pet.

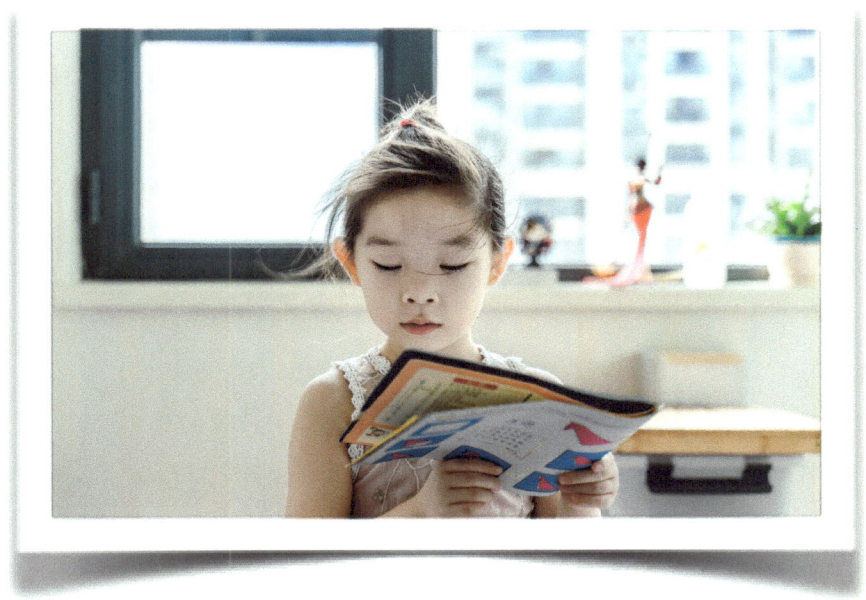

NEWSLETTER & BLOGS

Begin writing informative Laser therapy articles to insert into your newsletter. If you don't currently have a newsletter, start one!

You can highlight one benefit of Laser therapy or a case study in each issue of your newsletter that you can leave in your waiting room and /or send home at discharge.

Clients may also start to ask you questions about Laser therapy, which you may want to include in your newsletter. Be sure to obtain their permission to use their question(s). Many clients will be thrilled to know that they were able to influence your newsletter.

Blogs are another great way to reach your audience. Many website hosting software includes a blog page that can be easily inserted into your website.

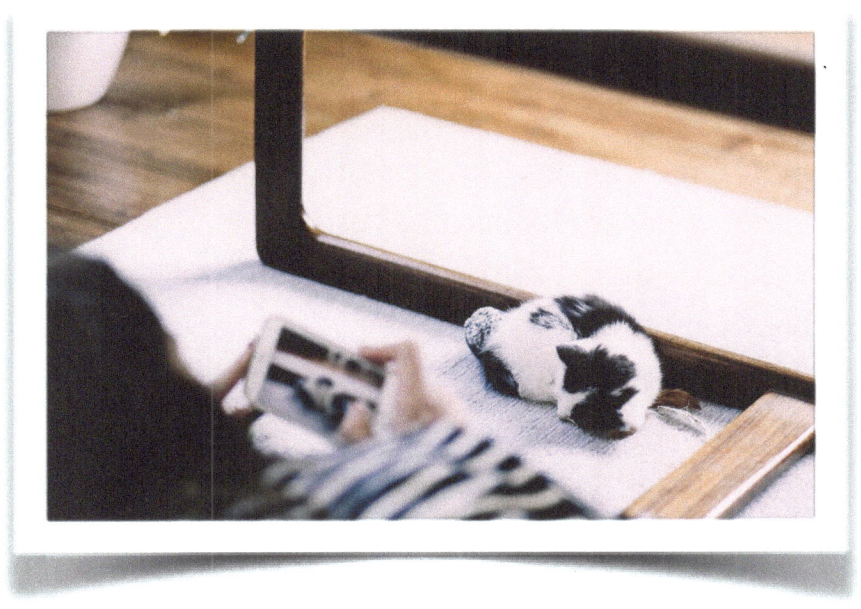

CASE STUDIES & TESTIMONIALS

Highlight interesting case studies to showcase on your own website. Get in the habit of taking before and after pictures along with videos. Live action video featuring a patient who can't walk - followed by post-Laser video showing the same patient who can now walk - is a powerful testament for renting your Laser (you must obtain the clients permission before posting or publishing them).

As you begin to see great results from your rental or Laser treatments, start asking for testimonials and receive their permission to use them on your website & brochures.

There are many different consent forms for both print, video and pictures. You can search the internet for samples and many can be downloaded for free. Here is one sample.

PET PHOTO CONSENT FORM

I, _____, hereby grant _____ permission to use any photographs taken of myself or my pet, in any and all of its publications, including website entries, without payment or any other consideration. I understand and agree that these materials will become your property and will not be returned. I hereby authorize to edit, alter, copy, exhibit, publish or distribute this photo for purposes of publicizing your programs or for any other lawful purpose.

In addition, I waive any right to royalties or other compensation arising or related to the use of the photograph. I hereby release rights to all claims, demands, and causes to action which I, my heirs, representatives, executors, administrators, or any other persons acting on my behalf of my estate have or may have by reason of this authorization. In signing this consent, I give authorization to use my name and my pet's name and information as printed below.

_____
(Pet's printed name)

_____   _____
(Owner's Signature)   (Date)

_____
(Owner's printed name)

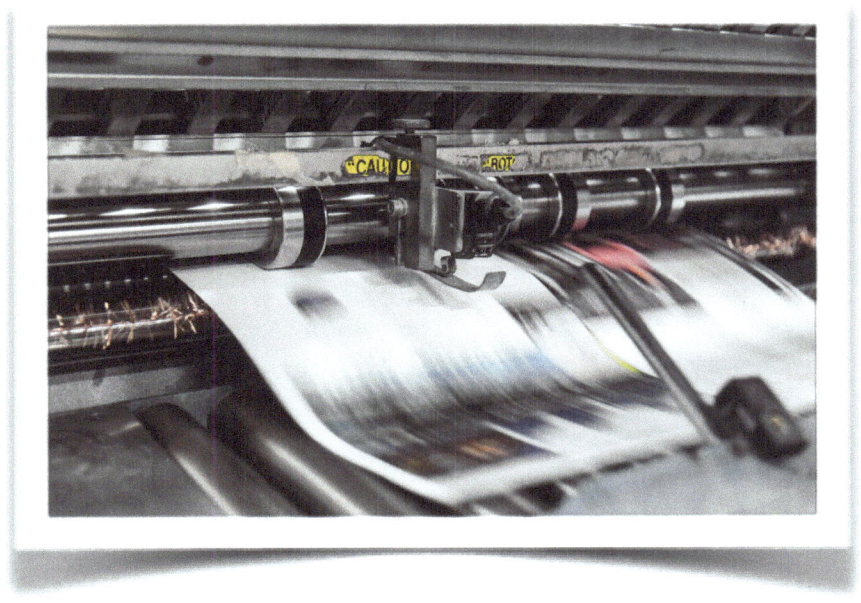

SUBMIT A PRESS RELEASE

Use a standard press release format to announce your new technology service to local media sources such as newspapers, radio and television stations.

On slow news days, you may be contacted by the producer or news reporter for an interview by the media. Make the heading of your press release timely and news worthy to what is currently happening, so timing is key to being selected.

For example, during Co-vid times, it is the perfect time to announce your rental Lasers that gives pets pain relief in the comfort of their own home. They can achieve pain relief with a no-touch and social distancing method since you can mail the disinfected Laser directly to the client.

You can also let them know that you use Teleconferencing to offer guidance and instructions on the use of the Laser, without having to be there.

Sample press releases can be found with the marketing materials provided with your MRM Lasers or you can also search for templates on the internet to download for free.

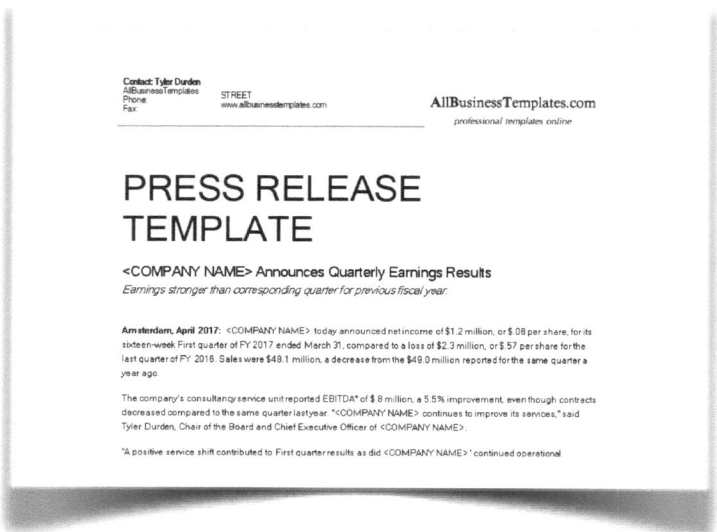

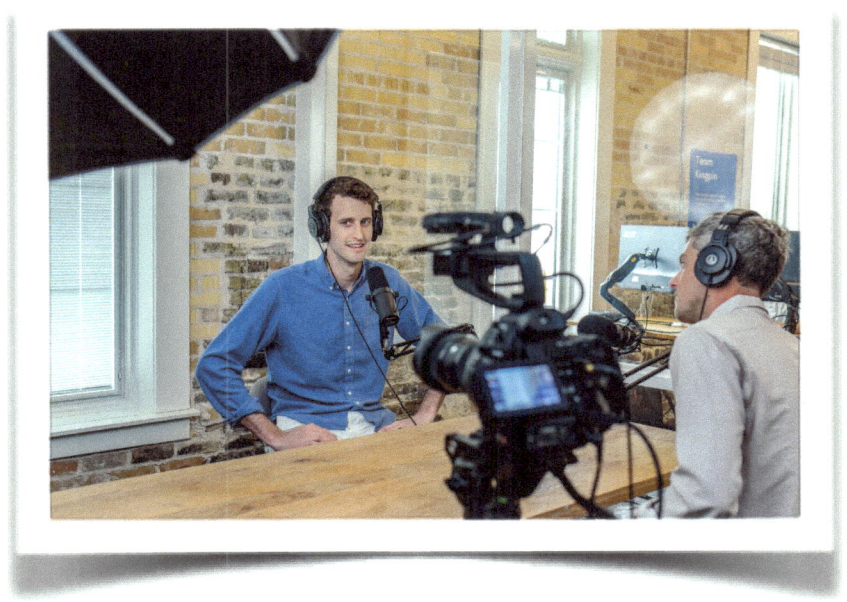

CONTACT YOUR LOCAL RADIO & TV STATIONS

Armed with your timely press release, contact the producers of your local radio or TV stations. Reporters and radio talk show hosts are always looking for engaging guests to appear on their program.

The more your story aligns with what is currently occurring in the news, the more likely you will be invited to be on air!

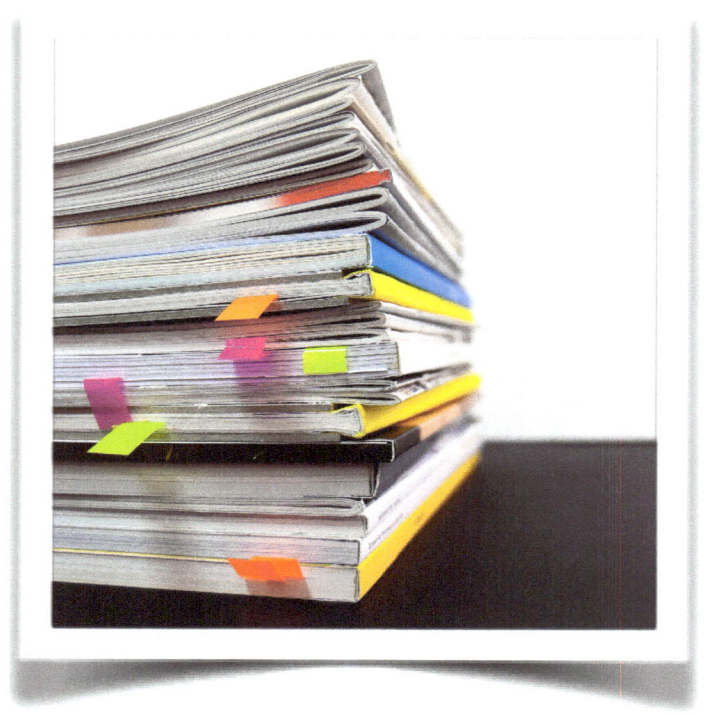

WRITE COLUMNS & ARTICLES

Contact the publishers of magazines & newspapers and inquire about writing a regular column or submitting an article for them. They will want to see samples of the type of articles you will write, and the most commonly accepted columns are the pet question and answer section.

It does not only have to be a pet related magazines such as Dogster and Catster. Articles can be submitted to Parenting type of publications and even weekly newsletters like Tidbits. Local area magazines are also a great place to feature your articles or columns.

The most important aspect of writing a column is meeting the publishers deadline, use their desired format and keep it right near their word count (but not over). Always submit by the deadline (if not before) to ensure that your section will be included in the next issue. The easier you make it for your publisher, the higher probability that you will become a regular columnist for their publication.

Remember that most magazines are 3 months ahead, so your questions should also reflect the season that the magazines will be out for distribution.

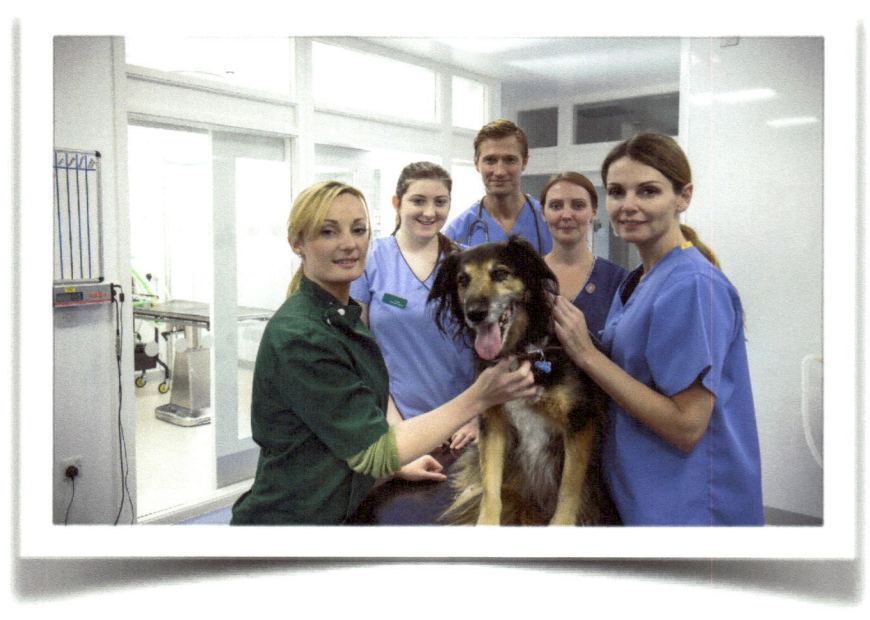

STAFF ENTHUSIASM!

Did you know that your staff & team is the most valuable asset for marketing your Lasers? They are the ones who talks to the clients at length and when they believe in the benefits of Laser Therapy, the team can boost your Laser therapy revenue!

Have you team feel the full benefit of the Laser on themselves. Try these Lasers for sore backs, necks, wrists and a variety of aches & pains.

When they feel the pain relief without using traditional drugs, they will be your biggest advocate for this modality.

But, if you don't want your team using these Lasers during work, try the Pain Pizza Game.

This is how you play this game:

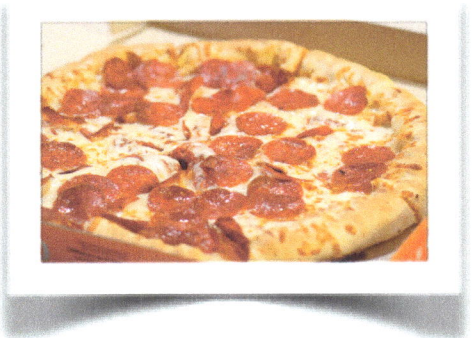

Use a bowl like a fishbowl or other container that team members can put money in. Name it the Pain Pizza Pot. Every time a team member needs to use the Laser, they must put money (you determine the amount) into the pot. Then they can Laser for 5 minutes during their break or after hours (this is the treatment time required for the MRM Laser to reduce pain). Once there is enough money in the pot to buy a pizza for the entire team, celebrate with a pain pizza lunch!

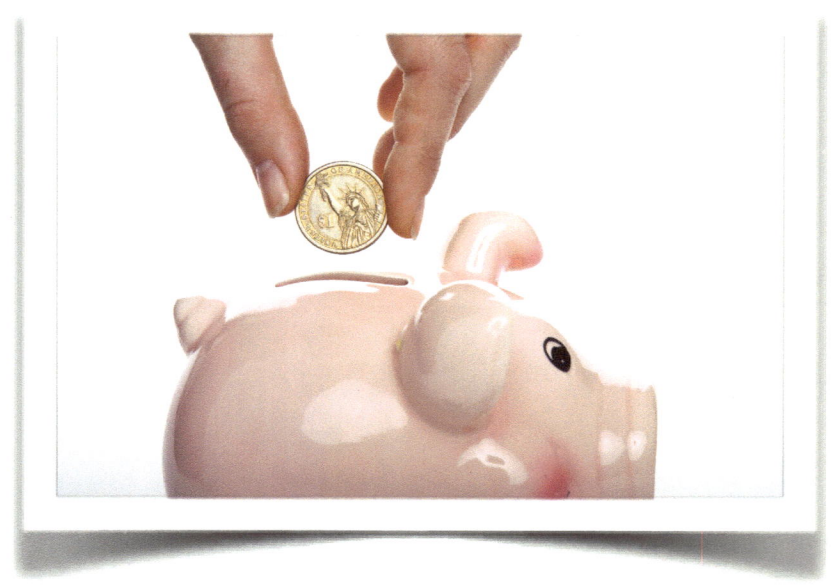

CREATE DISCOUNT PACKAGES

To make the rental packages more affordable, create discount packages. If you normally charge $50 for a Laser Therapy treatment in-house, you can give bundle discount such as 10% off a package of 6 sessions. Alternatively offer a deal where the client purchases 5 treatments and receives one free.

Then to make renting a Laser even more enticing, reduce the rental Laser for a week to be slightly less than or equal to the treatment that they would have to pay for in-house treatments. The owners can see for themselves that the rental option is more affordable if they have multiple pets at home (including themselves) that can benefit from Laser therapy treatments.

Additionally, many physicians have found that the client wants to continue to rent the Laser, even after their pet no longer feels pain. This is usually because human patients takes longer for the pain to subside. Continue to rent the Laser or sell them the Laser. I will address the profitable Affiliate Partnership program in another chapter.

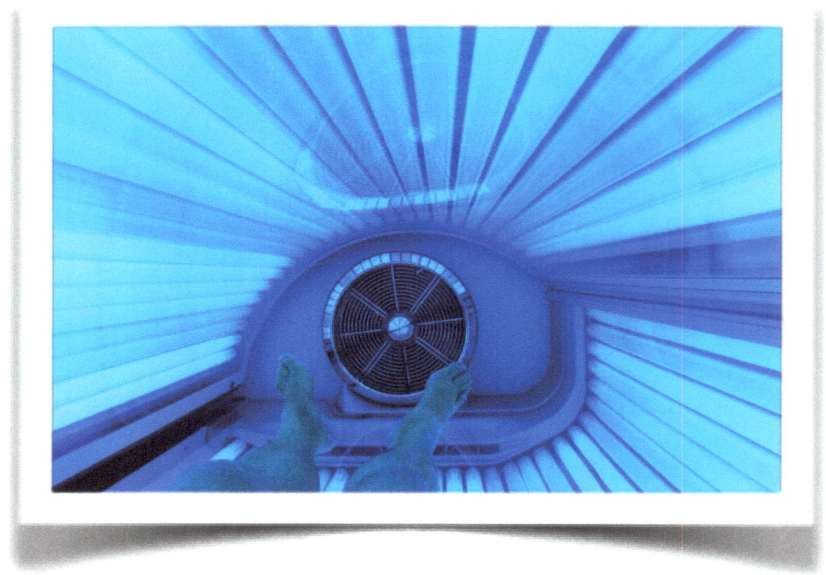

IN-HOUSE RENTALS

If you do not have enough rental Lasers or if you do not wish the Laser to leave the hospital, physicians are also offering in-house rentals much like tanning beds.

This plan works like this: clients will purchase a bundle of in-house rentals such as 6 sessions. The price of theses sessions are less than the cost of having a staff member or doctor to administer the Laser treatment.

Use a quiet exam room and show the client how to use the Laser on their pet the first time. For the next successive sessions, the clients will make an appointment to come in and Laser themselves. For example, Mrs Jones will come in at 1:00 pm. The Mr. Smith will come in at 1:10 pm. The sessions are usually less than 5 minutes long and you have time to clean the room and Laser between patients.

The beauty of this plan is that the Laser never leaves your facility, more clients are able to use the Laser and this method frees up your staff. Best of all, the pet receives the pain relief.

This method is not recommended for aggressive or fearful pets so please assess the pet & owner before recommending this option.

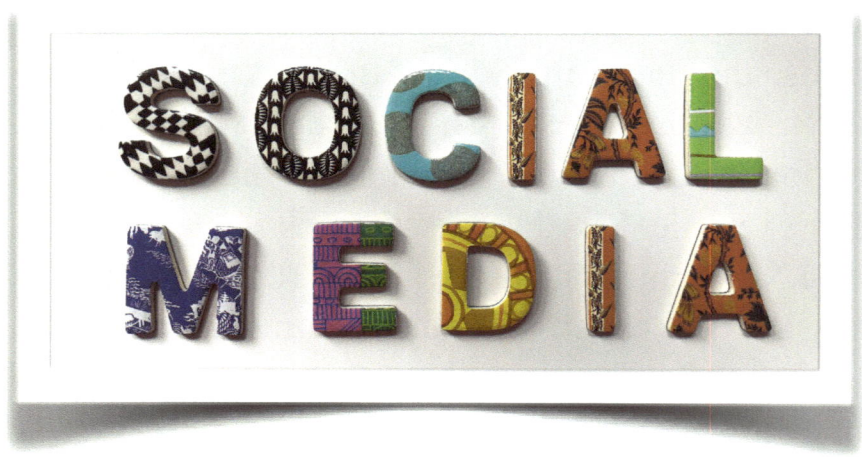

SOCIAL MEDIA POSTINGS

Social media presence is paramount in today's marketing plan. Whether it is a Facebook business page, your own You Tube channel, Instagram, Twitter, Yelp or other platforms, the very minimum you need is a website for your business.

There are now many do-it-yourself website hosting businesses. They have simple drag and drop software to build your website such as Vistaprint that has easy to use templates and will also obtain your domain name for you. Wix is another popular one with more features such as shopping carts and analytics but you will pay for each additional feature. GoDaddy has been around for a long time, but some people have reported that their website is not as user friendly as others. Not only can you obtain a domain name with GoDaddy but they also host your website for you. Search the internet for a variety of website building and hosting options available.

You can also hire a professional website hosting developer of which there are many. Whichever you choose, you still need to have a website for your business to have an internet presence.

You could spend hours and hours trying to post regularly on different social media channels or use a program that will automatically schedule to post your single message to many platforms at the same time.

SEO (Search Engine Optimization) is also another important factor to consider - to make sure that your business pops up on the first page of a search engine. There are many companies available that specialize in SEO and their service rate & contracts varies - so shop around. There are many good books, ebooks, videos and instructions available to teach you how to get the most out of social media postings.

This booklet does not cover all the nuances of social media as it is an entire lecture in itself. You can sign up to take courses on how to profit using social media. So please explore your options if you want to succeed in this ever-changing field of social media.

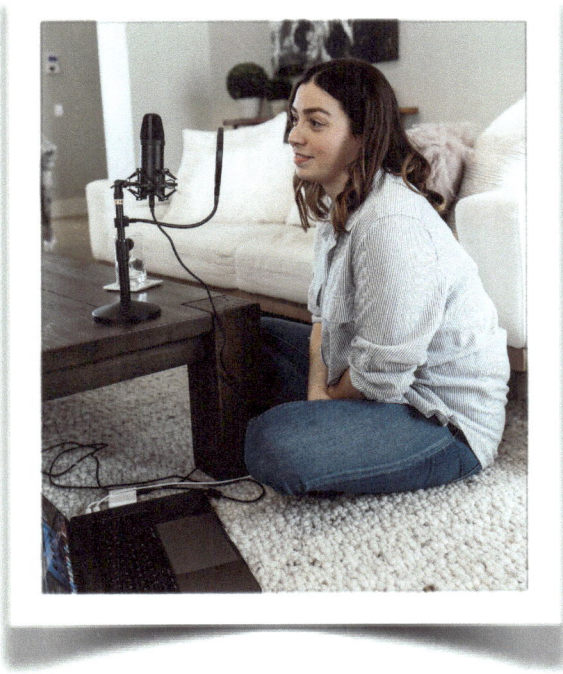

WEBINARS & PODCASTS

As more people turn to the internet for information, both webinars and podcasts have boomed in popularity.

There are many ways to create both. It can be as economical as using various free podcast creation apps available on both IOS or Android platforms such as Anchor. Some apps features the ability to distribute the finished recording to many podcast platforms at the same time.

You can also create webinars using your video phone and a quiet room. You don't need expensive equipment to produce & record a webinar. Others invest in editing software along with lots of hardware such as lighting, boom, microphones, backdrops and the list is endless, depending on the level of professionalism desired.

Live webinars are trickier as anything can happen during the broadcast. This can include computer glitches, loss of internet connection, unexpected visitors into your field of view and even stage fright! There is an appeal to live broadcasts but many viewers have a difficult time attending as life has a way of getting in the way of a perfectly planned schedule. In addition, there are currently multiple webinars being presented at the same time. It would be ideal to record the session to make it available for viewers at a later time.

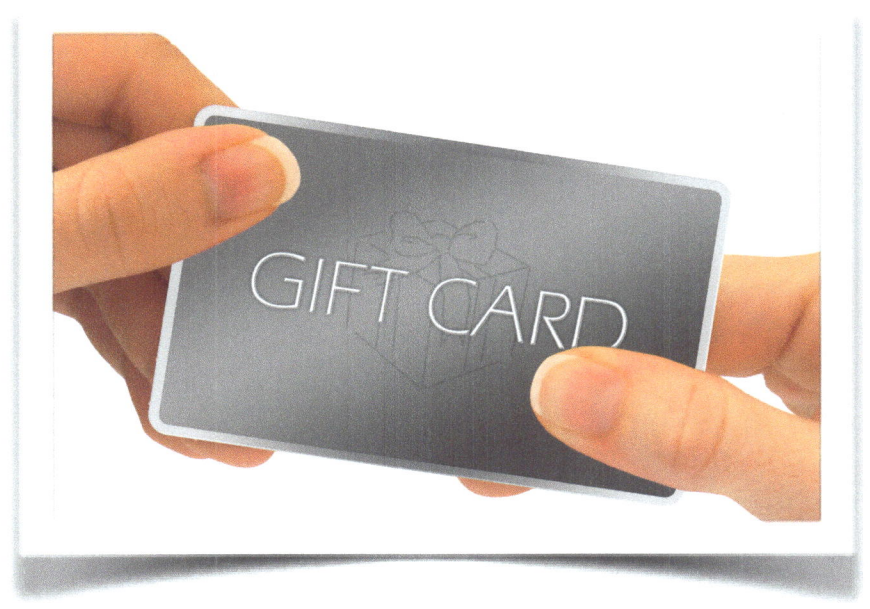

INCENTIVES & REFERRALS

In-house incentives can boost your team's willingness to sign clients up for rental Lasers. Create a plan that encourages your team members and rewards them with some sort of prize for each rental commitment. It can be as simple as a point system where once they reach a certain number of points, they win a prize or gift card. Don't make it competitive which harbors ill will and creates a hostile work environment. But rather, a joyous event for anyone who reaches that goal of the prize.

Some hospitals have instituted a small stipend for each rental contract completed. Whatever your prize is, the idea is to have your staff recommend the at-home Lasers to your clients.

You can also recruit referrals from your current rental clients. Ask them to recommend someone they know whose pet may benefit from the at-home treatments. If their referral results in a rental commitment, then reward them with a gift card or perhaps a free day of rental, etc.

Another idea would be a contest among renting clients. Place on your bulletin board or post on your website, pictures of their pets receiving Laser treatments at home. The winner every month receives some sort of prize and clients usually love to see their pets being showcased and highlighted at the clinic or website.

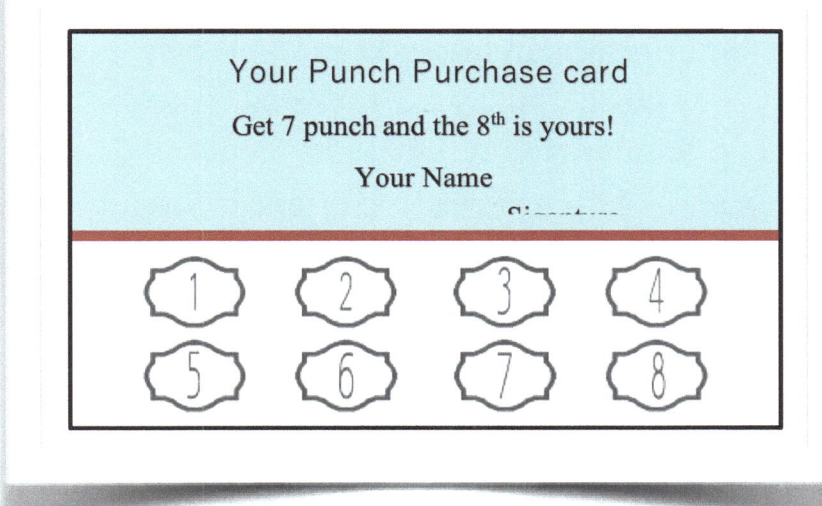

LOYALTY CARD

For your clients who rents frequently, you may want to start a punch card to reward them when this card is completed.

Create a business card with your information on the front and areas on the back which can keep track of their rentals. Some offices uses an unusual stamp or sticker to mark the card with completed rentals. Clients holding onto the card will continue to advertise your hospital and keep them as loyal rental clients.

You can also arm your team members with these cards with one square already marked off. This way, your staff can pass out these cards to prospective clients that they may meet outside of the hospital. The prospective client is already one rental closer to their prize!

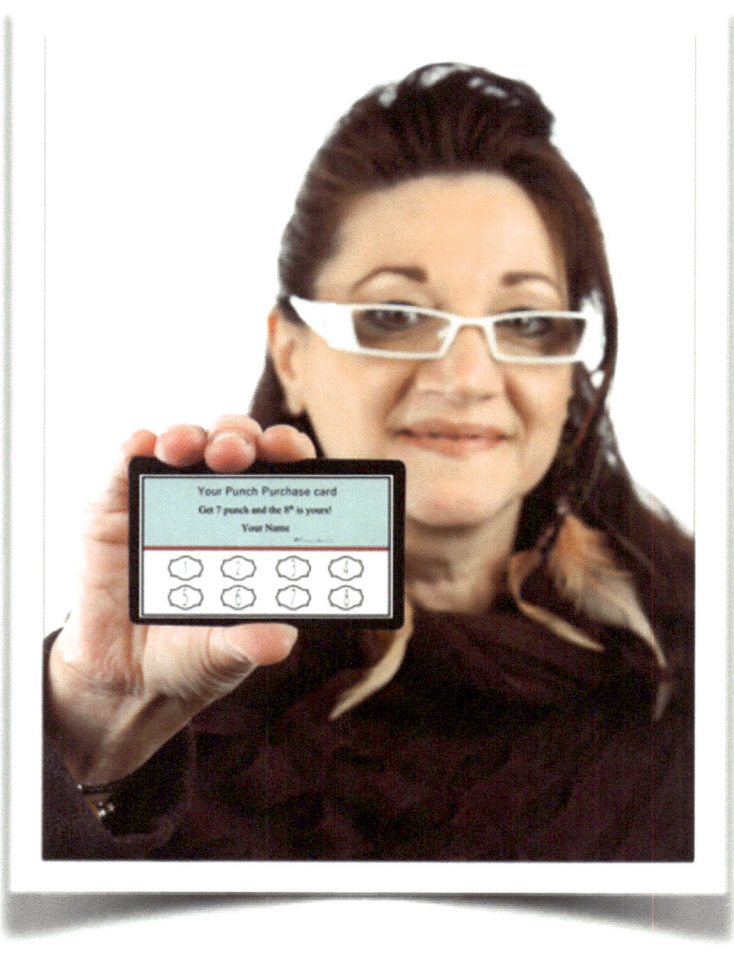

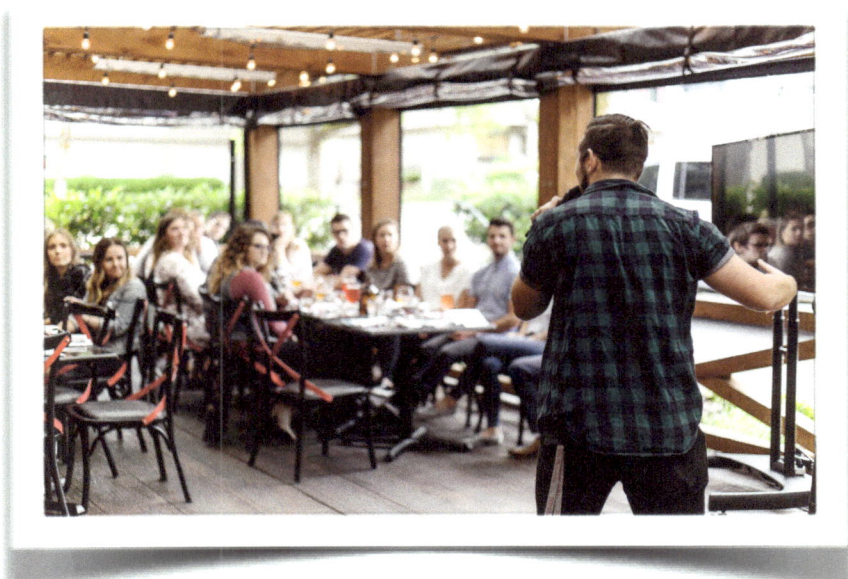

SPEAK AT LOCAL VENUES

Become an authority in your area by seeking out venues to speak. This could be senior centers, adult education courses, chamber of commerce events, churches, hobby groups, pet expos, pet fairs, etc.

Your presentation does not have to be long (10 - 15 minutes), but you can stand out as an authority in your area as the doctor who offers at-home rentals. This is also an opportune time to hand out your brochures and business cards.

You may even want to have a booth at these events. Your local pet expo and other neighborhood festivals often have booth sponsorship available. When you offer to speak in conjunction with your booth, sometimes the venue may give you a break in the cost of the booth itself.

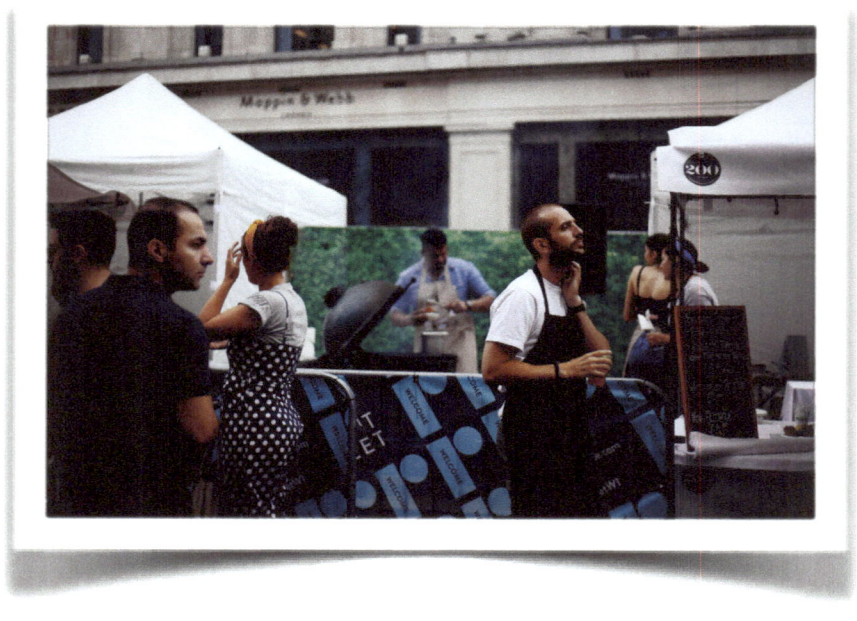

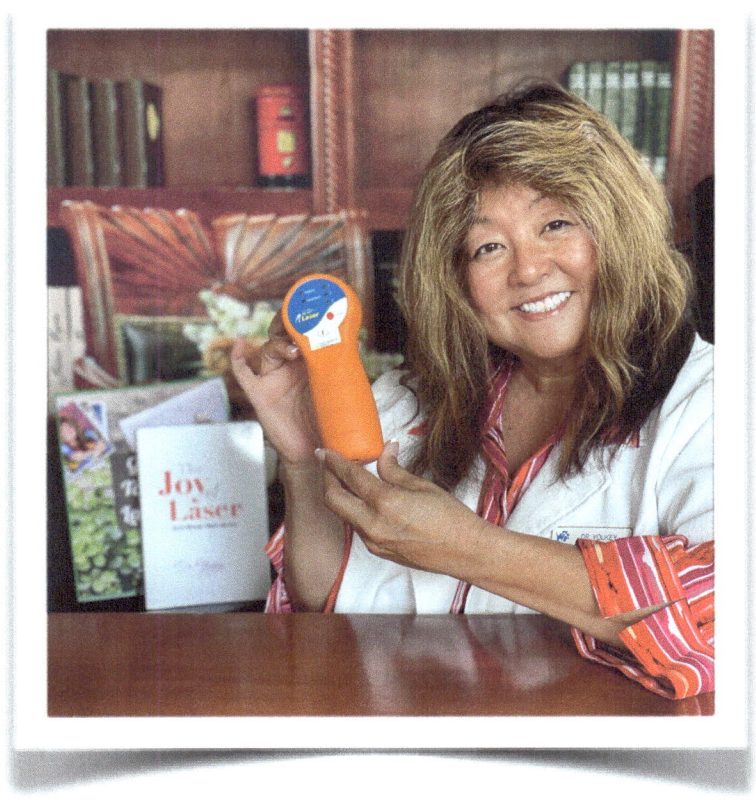

AFFILIATE PARTNERSHIP

There will come a time when your clients will want to purchase their own Laser. This is especially so when their pets will need a Laser for long term chronic conditions that will need continual treatments.

Instead of having your clients go on the internet and purchase a cheap imitation that is not FDA cleared or not approved for use in the USA, Dr. Youkey is offering you an option to sell a Laser directly to your clients with proven results.

You can also sell your rental Laser and obtain a replacement Laser at a lower price when you are a Affiliate Partner.

This is not an MLM (Multi Level Marketing). It is simply a way to partner with Dr. Youkey to be able to obtain Lasers at a lower cost - which can be drop-shipped directly to your client.

Please contact Dr. Youkey for more information if you would like to become an Affiliate Partner at dryoukey@mac.com.

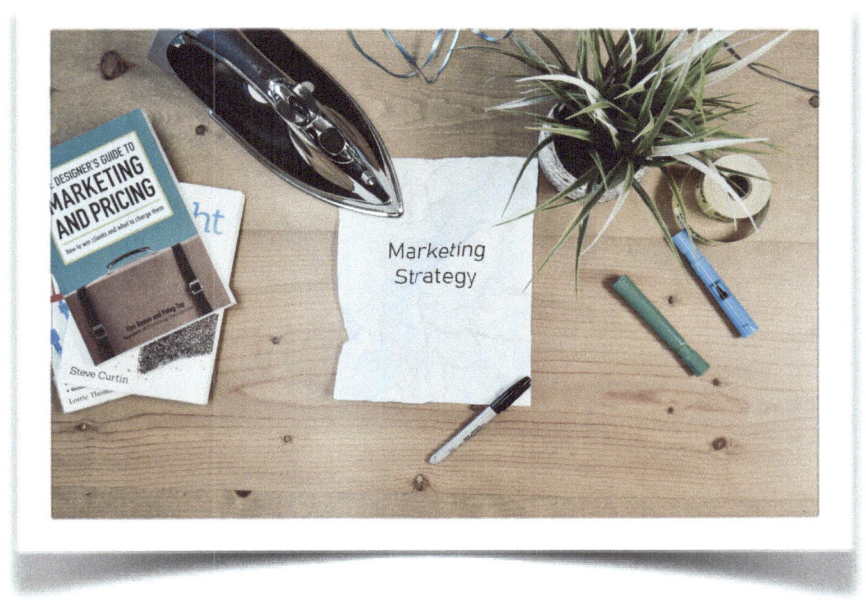

WANT MORE MARKETING TIPS?

This booklet was created to help you jump start your Laser rental service and filled with tips that have been used to promote Lasers in many practices.

Obviously this is not a complete list of ideas to help promote your new Laser service. There are many more marketing tips available at your local library, bookstore or the internet.

There are also Laser therapy tips available on the Facebook Blog: Cold Laser Therapy For Pets & People.

https://www.facebook.com/pg/coldlasertherapyforpetsandpeople/posts/?ref=page_internal

But with a little creative thinking and your teams enthusiasm, Laser therapy will become a very significant revenue generator for your practice.

Be sure to advertise that your practice uses the latest most effective and SAFE technology that is FDA cleared and approved for use in the USA!

Thank you for helping the pets enjoy a healthy pain-free life with at-home Lasers!

BONUS OFFER

As promised, this gift can be used toward your next Laser investment with Dr. Youkey. Please contact her at dryoukey@mac.com for the restrictions of this offer.

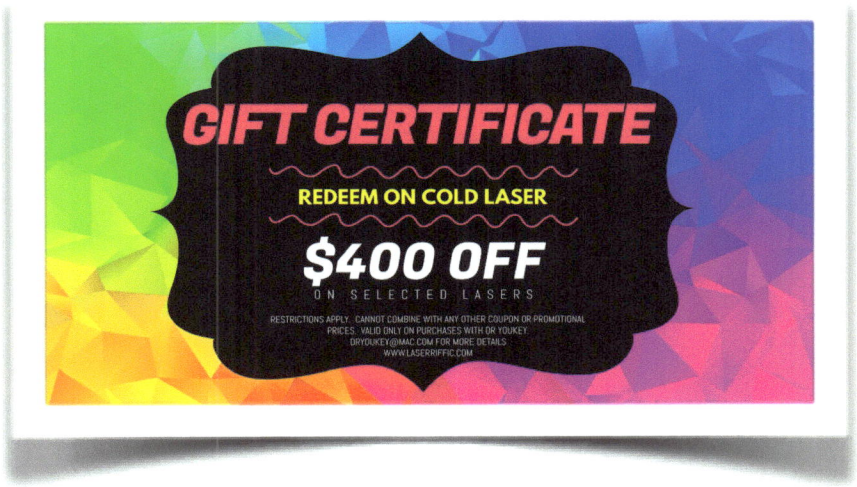

CONTACT INFORMATION

Email: dryoukey@mac.com

Website: www.laserriffic.com

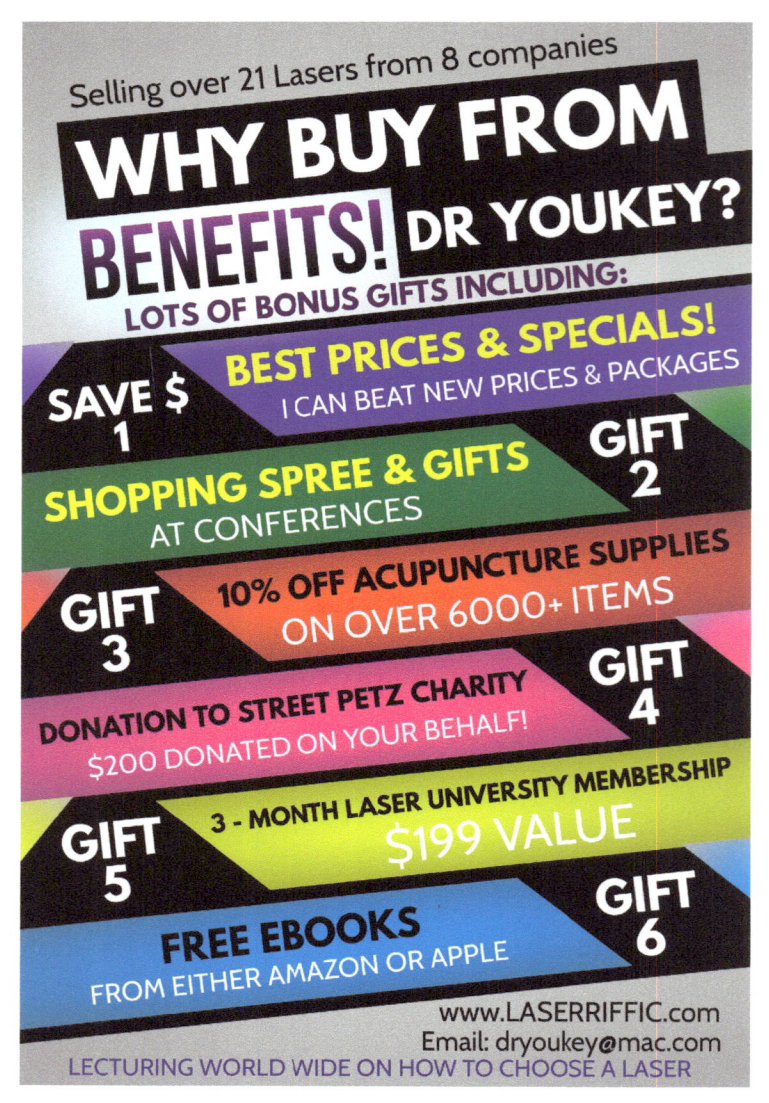

www.ingramcontent.com/pod-product-compliance
Lightning Source LLC
Chambersburg PA
CBHW040233220526
45473CB00001B/218